Hoodia

Weight-loss Wonder

Second Edition,
Revised and Updated

Editors of
Woodland Publishing

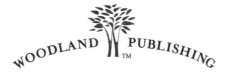

For order information, including bulk order discounts, and other inquiries, please contact:
Woodland Publishing
448 East 800 North
Orem, Utah 84097

Visit our Web site: www.woodlandpublishing.com
Call toll free: (800) 777-2665

ISBN: 978-1-58054-448-1

Contents

MOST OF US HAVE SEEN THE OLD-TIME MOVIES and cartoons set in the American West with raggedly dressed, parched, and near-dying men crawling across the sun-scorched sand. Minus a canteen—and probably food for that matter—they suddenly spot a lone cactus. Crawling to it, they barely have enough strength to cut into it, when voilà!—water pours out. They greedily drink and jump to their feet in no time. (Miraculously, many of them are also suddenly clean shaven.)

If only those suffering cowboys knew what an indigenous tribe halfway around the world has known for centuries, they could have avoided their suffering. In parts of Africa there are other deserts with different types of cactus-like plants. In these deserts, Kalahari Bushmen long ago discovered parts of a particular plant—*Hoodia gordonii*—that can yield more than just lifesaving liquid. For centuries now, they have eaten bite-size chunks to not only ward off thirst but to curb their appetites and eliminate hunger during long hunting trips in the wilderness.

And no wonder. Not only is there no running water in the Kalahari, there is virtually no surface water for most of the year. Only during the brief rainy season do the Bushmen—the most ancient group of nomadic hunter-gatherers on earth, and known to anthropologists as the San—have the luxury of a water supply. To survive during the rest of the year, they must rely on the water content of their food, the morning dew they collect from leaves, and the moisture they extract from other sources, such as underground tubers.

Besides thirst, the Bushman also learned how to suppress their appetite, an important survival skill in a region where just finding enough food to eat is a never-ending challenge, especially while on a lengthy hunt, when they walk or run as much as a hundred miles in pursuit of elusive prey. They realized that carrying food from home would slow them down. Then, once they killed their prey, they needed to avoid temptation and not eat any of it before carrying it home to share equally with everyone in the village. To escape their distress from unending hunger pangs they'd chew on *Hoodia gordonii*.

In an interview with ABC News in 2003, Andries Steenkamp, a spokesman for the San people, said, "I learned how to eat it from my forefathers. It is my food, my water, and also a medicine for me. We San use the plant during hunting to fight off the pain of hunger and thirst."

Although it looks like a small cactus, *Hoodia gordonii*—commonly known as hoodia—is actually a type of milkweed. It thrives in very high temperatures and takes years to mature.

Since hoodia is a succulent, it contains a good deal of moisture. Although bitter tasting, it is a welcome relief when you have few if any alternatives in the desert. Sucking on the pulpy flesh, the Bushmen could not only quell their thirst but also ward off their hunger. In addition, according to Bushman lore, hoodia gives them enough energy to walk all day or make love all night, plus it cures a hangover and settles an upset stomach.

Hoodia Comes West

Film buffs may remember the Bushmen in the movie *The Gods Must Be Crazy*. Although the West is just discovering hoodia, the Bushmen of the Kalahari, who have been living off the land in southern Africa for thousands of years, have been eating it for a very long time.

The first supplements containing the hoodia compound were introduced in the United States in early 2004 to aid in obesity and weight loss by suppressing appetite. Thus, hoodia became one of the newest entries in the crowded weight-loss sweepstakes.

The U.S. market for an effective weight-loss remedy is huge. Being overweight is the most common chronic disease risk factor in the United States, with more than 50 percent of the U.S. population being overweight. The number of overweight people has increased rapidly among all segments of the population, and the trend is expected to continue. Obesity doesn't just make it hard to fit into your clothes. Obesity increases risk of chronic diseases and conditions including:

• High blood pressure
• High cholesterol

- Type 2 diabetes
- Coronary artery disease
- Stroke
- Gallbladder disease
- Osteoarthritis
- Sleep apnea
- Respiratory problems
- Endometrial, breast, prostate, and colon cancers

Specifically, the Centers for Disease Control and Prevention (CDC) report that the 1990s witnessed dramatic increases in the incidence of diabetes and obesity in the United States; and at the same time, Americans showed little improvement in eating habits or in increasing their physical activity.

In a study recently published in the *Journal of the American Medical Association (JAMA)*, the CDC found a 61 percent increase in the percentage of obese Americans from 1991 to 2000 and a 49 percent increase in the percentage of Americans with diabetes.

More alarming, the rate of obesity among children has increased dramatically in the past two decades. With it, some formerly rare health problems such as high cholesterol, high blood pressure, and type 2 diabetes are becoming more common among the young.

If people could lose weight simply by popping a pill or capsule, all the better. It's estimated that each year, people spend more than $40 billion on products designed to help them slim down.

Why Do We Eat So Much?

It's easy to blame it simply on a lack of self-control. While to some degree that's true, at no other time in the history of our species have we lived in an environment of such tremendous food availability and the marketing savvy to pique your interest.

Not only is food pretty much there for the asking on every street corner, but it is also highly processed and refined. You simply could not get super-sized french fries and a chocolate shake in 1905 the way you can in 2005. Or in the African desert in any year, for that matter. Today food portions in the United States are huge, and most people think processed food tastes better than it does in its natural state—sweeter, smoother, and less chewy—and the caloric content is higher. Even "natural" foods like grapes are subject to cross-breeding to produce a finished "product" with very high sugar content.

Some of us have a genetic make-up that can handle environments of high food availability. These individuals have genes that "know" that food is always around, that there is no need to store extra calories as fat; and they have a higher basal metabolic rate, or a continually lower appetite, to remain thin.

The rest of us, however, have genes that harken back to our roots and are constantly worried about the coming winter, when food will be scarce, the food shelves will be bare, and there will only be a few leftover potatoes and carrots to ration. These genes command our bodies to eat more food and store the extra as fat for the coming winter. Of course, when the barren winter never comes, the fat we store doesn't get burned and we get more and more overweight.

What Is Hoodia?

Hoodia gordonii is a succulent plant belonging to the milkweed (Asclepiadaceae) family that consists of approximately twenty species. Known in the Kalahari as xhoba, hoodia is a leafless, spiny plant—not truly a cactus—with fleshy finger-like stems. There are rows of thorns along the stems, and the plants bear flesh-colored flowers. The strong smell of decaying meat attracts flies to the flowers, which lay their eggs inside and pollinate them.

Sometimes it is spelled hootia, hodia, hoodie, and hudia. Recently, hoodia garnered a great deal of attention after being featured on CBS' *60 Minutes* and the BBC in the United Kingdom.

Hoodia grows in summer rainfall areas in Angola, Botswana, Namibia, and South Africa, as well as winter rainfall areas in Namibia. Only one species is found east of 26 degrees longitude, (*H. currorii subsp. Lugardii*), which appears in Botswana and the Limpopo province of South Africa. Although the genus Hoodia is widespread in southern Africa, *Hoodia gordonii* only grows in South Africa and Namibia despite some claims to the contrary. *Hoodia gordonii* is the only species that contains the chemical component that suppresses appetite. For the rest of this booklet, "hoodia" will refer specifically to *Hoodia gordonii*.

As I've already said, for thousands of years, hoodia has been used by San Bushmen populating the arid territories of South Africa and Namibia. Since they needed to remain active to survive, they had little need to diet, but learned that this plant provided stamina and curbed hunger during prolonged periods without food. Besides the benefit of reducing or eliminating the desire for food, many believe hoodia also increases energy and can have an aphrodisiac effect on the user.

Hoodia's appetite-suppressing ingredient is a molecule similar to glucose, only stronger. The Council for Scientific and Industrial Research (CSIR) in South Africa isolated an active compound for appetite suppression from hoodia known as P57, which seems to send a signal to the hypothalamus of the brain and "tricks" the body into believing it is no longer hungry. The result is a complete lack of appetite.

Among the many chemical compounds found in the sap of hoodia, scientists in South Africa have discovered an appetite-suppressing compound with a long and complicated name they've dubbed P57. P57 is a steroidal glycoside, a steroid molecule chemically bonded to a chain of three sugar molecules.

Some years back, scientists at Brown University Medical School in Providence, Rhode Island, became interested in P57 as a means for investigating how the sense of satiety, or fullness, is induced in our brains, telling us to stop eating. Because P57 is an anorectic (an agent that suppresses appetite), they believed pinpointing the mechanism by which it acts on the brain should shed some light on this question. They found the appetite-suppressing and mood-enhancing property (ten thousand times as active as glucose) goes to the mid-brain causing neuron cells to fire as if you were full—even when you're not.

Additional interest in hoodia cropped up a few years ago when it was revealed that Pfizer, the pharmaceutical company, planned to introduce a new diet drug made from the plant. Pfizer subsequently stopped its research into the plant, but the ensuing publicity, and now the *60 Minutes* coverage, has caused a surge in interest in this "new" botanical remedy for obesity—joining a slew of other supplements and prescription diet pills in an increasingly crowded field after the Food and Drug Administration (FDA) banned ephedra.

Hoodia is very different from ephedra and the banned diet drug combination fen-phen because hoodia isn't a stimulant. Scientists say it fools the brain by making you think you're full, even if you've eaten just a morsel.

How Does It Work?

The hypothalamus is the region of the brain that contains several important centers that control body temperature, thirst, hunger, water balance, and sexual function. The hypothalamus is also closely connected with emotional activity and sleep, and functions as a center for the integration of hormonal and autonomic nervous activity through its control of pituitary secretions. The hypothalamus links the nervous system to the endocrine system.

In our bodies, the pituitary gland is often portrayed as the "master gland," since the anterior and posterior pituitary secrete a battery of hormones that collectively influence all cells and affect virtually all physiological processes. However, the power behind the pituitary gland is the hypothalamus, because some of the neurons within the hypothalamus—neurosecretory neurons—secrete hormones that strictly control the secretion of hormones from the anterior pituitary. The hypothalamic hormones are referred to as releasing hormones and inhibiting hormones, reflecting their influence on anterior pituitary hormones.

Hypothalamic releasing and inhibiting hormones are carried directly to the anterior pituitary gland via hypothalamic-hypophyseal portal veins. Here, hypothalamic hormones bind to receptors on anterior pituitary cells, modulating the release of the hormone they produce.

The P57 compound found in hoodia appears to work by increasing the content of adenosine triphosphate (ATP) in nerve cells in the hypothalamus. ATP is an energy-producing molecule formed from glucose, the brain's favorite fuel source. When levels of ATP are increased in hypothalamic nerve cells, it appears that those nerve cells fire as if you had just eaten, even when you haven't.

Under Study

In the 1960s, the Bushmen disclosed the use of hoodia for appetite suppression to the South African army. The Pretoria-based CSIR then undertook animal studies with hoodia in the 1980s. The first scientific investigation of the plant was conducted at the CSIR, a partially state-funded laboratory in South Africa. Because Bushmen were known to eat hoodia, it was included in a study of indigenous foods.

Still the how and why of hoodia's use as an appetite suppressant wasn't immediately recognized. In fact, it took the laboratory thirty years to isolate and identify the specific appetite-suppressing ingredient in hoodia. "It took them a long time," said Dr. Richard Dixey during the *60 Minutes* broadcast. "In fact, the original research was done in the mid-1960s. What they found was when they fed it to animals, the animals ate it and lost weight."

Rights to CSIR's patent suite were then licensed to Phytopharm PLC, the U.K.-based botanical pharmaceutical company headed by Dixey. According to Dixey, the patent is on the active compounds within the plant and its use as a weight-loss material. "It's not on the plant itself," he said.

In 1998, Phytopharm signed a sublicensing agreement with Pfizer, allowing the pharmaceutical company to commercialize an obesity drug based on the hoodia compound. Five years later, Pfizer ended its relationship with Phytopharm. Phytopharm, which has established hoodia plantations worldwide to meet the expected demand, is now looking elsewhere for a licensing partner, based not just on P57 but also on numerous semisynthetic analogs of P57 that it has produced in the interim.

In the United States, scientists at Brown University Medical School were also intrigued by the fact that P57 is chemically similar to a class of plant-derived compounds called cardiac glycosides—with ones derived from various foxglove species the best known. These powerful drugs increase the force of contraction of the heart muscle and help maintain normal heart rate and rhythm. A common side effect of cardiac glycosides is loss of appetite.

Like many drugs, cardiac glycosides act by interacting with specific receptor molecules embedded in the walls of our cells. When stimulated by such interactions, these receptors, which are large, complex proteins that act as molecular channels, initiate a chain of events inside the cell. With cardiac glycosides, the receptor molecule is called Na/K-ATPase. Its primary function is to regulate the flow of sodium ions and potassium ions into and out of the cell through the molecular channel, using chemical energy provided by molecules of adenosine triphosphate (ATP). This process, called a sodium/potassium pump, is critically important in maintaining proper cell function and allowing cells to perform certain actions, such as muscle contraction—including the heart muscle—and nervous impulse transmission.

Despite the similarities—including the appetite-suppressing effect—between P57 and cardiac glycosides, initial studies with P57 failed to show any effect on Na/K-ATPase receptors, meaning P57 is probably not a cardiac glycoside. P57 also failed to show an effect on a wide range of other types of receptors. Thus its mode of action at the cellular level is something of a mystery.

How About Humans?

The first human clinical trial conducted by Phytopharm included a group of morbidly obese men and women chosen from Leicester, England, and placed in a prison-like "phase 1 unit". All the volunteers could do was read, watch television—and eat. Half the group was given hoodia and half was given a placebo. At the end of fifteen days, the group on hoodia had reduced their food intake by 1,000 calories a day. The average American man consumes about 2,600 calories a day; a woman about 1,900.

By the end of the study, those in the hoodia group had reduced their caloric intake by 30 percent, plus lost more than 2 pounds of pure body fat with no exercise—a couch potato's dream.

So far, Phytopharm has spent more than $20 million on research, including the clinical trials with obese volunteers that yielded promising results. "If you take this compound every day, your wish to eat goes down. And we've seen that very, very dramatically," said Dixey.

Research continues both in the United States and overseas. In two recent double-blind studies, Brown University researchers conducted experiments with normal, healthy rats in which they injected minuscule amounts of P57 directly into their brains—specifically, into a small cavity called the third intracerebral ventricle, located above the hypothalamus, which lies deep in the forebrain, just above the pituitary gland.

The purpose of these injections was to determine whether P57's appetite-suppressing effect is the result of its direct action on the hypothalamus. The researchers now believe it is. In these studies, lean and obese laboratory rats were given hoodia, which strongly suppressed their appetites and caused major weight loss in the obese rats and moderate appetite suppression and weight loss in the lean rats. Hoodia also induced a modest drop in the rats' blood-sugar levels, and no adverse side effects were reported.

Specifically, the researchers found food intake was reduced by 50 to 60 percent during the first twenty-four hours after the injections, and the effect, which was dose dependent, lasted for about twenty-four to forty-eight hours. These reductions in food intake were observed in comparison with that of a group of control rats, which had also had an inert substance injected into their brains. The researchers concluded that the reductions represented a genuine effect due to P57.

They also found that injections in the abdominal cavity (intraperitoneal) of P57 did not significantly reduce the rats' food intake. This suggests that, for it to work, P57 must enter the bloodstream, which carries it to all parts of the body, including the hypothalamus.

The Brown researchers conducted additional studies on cell cultures. These studies confirmed the lack of a direct effect of P57 on the Na/K-ATPase receptors in hypothalamic cell cultures. They did find, however, that P57 blocked the action of ouabain—a cardiac glycoside—on these receptors. Ouabain is a white poisonous glycoside extracted from the seeds of African trees used as a heart stimulant and by some African peoples as a dart poison.

The researchers ruled out a direct toxic effect since there has been no evidence of toxicity for P57, either in laboratory experiments or in animal studies. They decided to test for an effect of P57 on the intracellular concentration of ATP, the energy molecule that drives the sodium/potassium pump mentioned earlier.

Using a hypothalamic cell culture, they found that P57 increased the concentration of ATP by about 50 percent following a thirty-minute incubation (ouabain had no such effect). When they tested for a similar effect in live rats that were fed a normal diet, they found that brains injected with P57 had increased hypothalamic ATP levels by about 100 percent—more than two-fold—compared with the controls.

The researchers then tested rats that had been on a severe low-calorie diet for four days. Without P57, these rats had hypothalamic ATP levels about 40 percent below normal (the ATP levels in their livers were about 60 percent below normal). It is reasonable to expect such decreases, because ATP is created in the body by the metabolism of food, so less food should result in less ATP—unless some other factor temporarily stimulates increased production of ATP. And that, apparently, is what P57 did, at least in the hypothalamus: when these underfed rats were brain-injected with P57, their hypothalamic ATP levels rose to about normal, whereas the ATP levels in the control rats remained low.

In case this scientific discussion made your eyes glaze over, suffice it to say that increased ATP production is a biochemical signal that means that you've had enough food—therefore, you don't feel hungry, so you should stop eating.

The Brown University authors did offer one caveat. Their demonstration of P57's appetite-suppressing action in the central nervous system in no way precludes the possibility that it may act to suppress appetite in other ways in other parts of the body as well, possibly through effects on the peripheral nervous system, on the stomach, or on potentially appetite-suppressing hormones, such as CCK (cholecystokinin). CCK is a kind of naturally occurring appetite-suppressant chemical. As food is digested and your body's cells are "fed," CCK is released and your brain tells you to stop eating.

Some drug companies are developing CCK-booster supplements to reduce appetite in those who suffer from severe obesity. How effective these CCK boosters will be remains to be seen.

Hoodia and Diabetes

As mentioned in the paper by the Brown researchers, there have been several unpublished studies with rats and humans in which homogenates or extracts of hoodia produced substantial anorectic (appetite-suppressing) effects that lasted for the duration of the studies (up to eight weeks). Included in these studies were experiments with obese diabetic rats, in which hoodia was claimed to have produced a "reversal of diabetes." Although it's not clear to what extent this occurred (and there was no indication of the source of the information), any degree of reversal of diabetes is obviously desirable.

Another hint of such an effect came in two brief papers published a few years ago in which it was claimed that hoodia produced "modest decreases" in blood glucose 2 and a 15 percent decrease in blood glucose 3 in both lean and obese (but non-diabetic) rats. These improvements accompanied a substantial loss of weight in the rats, owing to hoodia's anorexic effect. It is well known that obesity and type 2 diabetes go hand in hand in humans and that weight loss in obese individuals tends to reverse the symptoms of diabetes. If hoodia can induce both weight loss and glucose reduction independently, as may be the case, so much the better.

Is Hoodia Safe?

Marketers of hoodia say the most compelling evidence for the safety and efficacy of *Hoodia gordonii* as an appetite suppressant comes from its use by the Bushmen of the Kalahari for thousands of years. Nonetheless, modern pharmacologists and physicians would like to see scientific evidence for the benefits of hoodia, if only to learn how it works and how, perhaps, it could be made to work even better. So far, there have been no published clinical trials on hoodia in peer-reviewed scientific journals, although there have been unpublished reports of its efficacy by two drug companies that have been developing it for commercial purposes.

Using Hoodia

Some people say hoodia works for them immediately, suppressing appetite within twenty to thirty minutes after taking the capsules. Generally, though, people typically need up to two weeks of regularly taking hoodia before they begin to notice its effects, which include:

- Reduced interest in food
- Delay in the time after eating before hunger returns
- More rapid onset of satiety
- General feeling of well-being

Controversy as an Added Ingredient

But what does that say about all these weight-loss products that claim to contain hoodia? Trimspa said its X32 pills contain 75 mg of hoodia. The company is marketing its product with an ad campaign featuring Anna Nicole Smith, even though the FDA has notified Trimspa that it hasn't demonstrated that the product is safe.

In the *60 Minutes* broadcast, coeditor and CBS News correspondent Lesley Stahl interviewed Dr. Dixey from Phytopharm, the U.K.-based research company that holds a patent on the use of a special hoodia extract for weight loss. Since many importers have introduced products that claim to contain hoodia, the *60 Minutes* segment covered issues of bio-piracy and royalty payments to the indigenous Kalahari Bushmen who have used hoodia for millennia.

Dr. Dixey claims some companies have even used the results of Phytopharm's clinical tests to market their products. "This is just straightforward theft. That's what it is. People are stealing data, which they haven't done, they've got no proper understanding of, and [are] sticking [it] on the bottle," Dr. Dixey told *60 Minutes*. "When we have assayed these materials, they contain between 0.1 and 0.01 percent of the active ingredient claimed. But they use the term hoodia on the bottle, of course, so they—does nothing at all."

But Dr. Dixey isn't the only one who has felt ripped off. The Bushmen first heard the news about the patent when Phytopharm put out a press release. Roger Chennells, an attorney in South Africa who represents the Bushmen—the San—was appalled.

"The San did not even know about it," said Chennells. "They had given the information that led directly toward the patent." Stahl pointed out that the taking of traditional knowledge without compensation is called "bio-piracy."

"You have said, and I'm going to quote you, 'that the San felt as if someone had stolen the family silver,'" said Stahl to Chennells. "So what did you do?"

"I wouldn't want to go into some of the details as to what kind of letters were written or what kind of threats were made," said Chennells. "We engaged them. They had done something wrong, and we wanted them to acknowledge it."

Chennells was determined to help the Bushmen who, he said, were exploited for centuries. First they were pushed aside by black tribes. Then, when white colonists arrived, they were nearly annihilated.

"About the turn of the century, there were still hunting parties in Namibia and in South Africa that allowed farmers to go and kill Bushmen," said Chennells. "It's well documented."

The Bushmen are still stigmatized in South Africa, and plagued with high unemployment, little education, and a high rate of alcoholism. And now, it seemed they were about to be cut out of a potential windfall from hoodia. So Chennells threatened to sue the national lab on their behalf.

"We knew that if it was successful, many, many millions of dollars would be coming towards the San," said Chennells. "Many, many millions. They've talked about the market being hundreds and hundreds of millions in America."

In the end, a settlement was reached—thanks to the legal efforts of various organizations acting on behalf of the San. In an unusual example of cross-cultural goodwill, an amicable benefit-sharing agreement was reached in 2003 whereby the San (of whom there are about one hundred thousand left) will be rewarded with 6 percent of all royalties received by the CSIR, and 8 percent of the CSIR's milestone income received when certain targets are reached.

Although this represents but a tiny slice of the pie (the CSIR's slice is small to begin with—probably about 10 percent of Phytopharm's royalties), that pie could turn out to be huge. The market potential for a safe and effective appetite suppressant could easily be in the billions annually—especially when pharmaceutical companies sell it at inflated prices as a prescription drug. Thus a good deal of money could soon befall the San, who until recently didn't even know what money was, and would have had no use for it in any case; most of them are still unclear about its purpose and value.

Free Publicity

Still, despite the controversy, in the crowded weight-loss field, it's very difficult to get the message out and distinguish a particular remedy—whether it works or not. Marketers of hoodia hit the jackpot when *60 Minutes* traveled to South Africa to investigate the attributes and claims about its weight-loss properties.

For the *60 Minutes* story, Nigel Crawhall, a linguist and interpreter, hired an experienced tracker named Toppies Kruiper, a local aboriginal Bushman, to help find some hoodia.

Kruiper led the *60 Minutes* crew out into the desert. When asked if he ate hoodia, Kruiper replied, speaking through an interpreter, "I really like to eat them when the new rains have come. Then they're really quite delicious."

After locating a plant, Kruiper cut off a stalk that resembled a small, spiky pickle, and removed the sharp spines. He offered a sample to Stahl. On camera, she described the taste as "a little cucumbery in texture, but not bad."

She then reported that it left no funny taste in her mouth, no queasy stomach, and no racing heart. She also noted that she wasn't hungry all day, even when she would normally have a pang around mealtime. And, she also had no desire to eat or drink the entire day. "I'd have to say it did work," said Stahl.

In a recent *BBC Two* report, correspondent Tom Mangold had a similar reaction. "The plant is said to have a feel-good almost aphrodisiac quality, and I have to say, we felt good," said Mangold. "But more significantly, we did not even think about food. Our brains really were telling us we were full. It was a magnificent deception.

Dinner time came and went. We reached our hotel at about midnight and went to bed without food. And the next day, neither of us wanted nor ate breakfast.

"I ate lunch but without appetite and very little pleasure. Partial then full appetite returned slowly after twenty-four hours."

Hoodia's Future

The future of hoodia is still uncertain. Further development of hoodia for weight loss hit a major snag last year. As mentioned previously, Pfizer, which had teamed up with Phytopharm and had funded much of the research, dropped the project when making a pill out of the active ingredient seemed out of reach.

Dixey said it can be made synthetically: "We've made milligrams of it. But it's very expensive. It's not possible to make it synthetically in what's called a scaleable process. So we couldn't make a metric ton of it or something that is the sort of quantity you'd need to actually start doing something about obesity in thousands of people."

Phytopharm decided to market hoodia in its natural form, in diet shakes and bars. That meant it needed the hoodia plant itself. But given the obesity epidemic in the United States and other countries, it became obvious that what was needed was a lot of hoodia— much more than was growing in the wild in the Kalahari. 60 Minutes visited one of Phytopharm's hoodia plantations in South Africa. Phytopharm says they'll need a lot of these plantations if demand meets their expectations.

Agronomist Simon MacWilliam has a tall order: grow a billion portions of hoodia a year, within just a couple of years. He admitted that starting up the plantation has been quite a challenge.

"The problem is we're dealing with a novel crop. It's a plant we've taken out of the wild and we're starting to grow it," said MacWilliam. "So we have no experience. So it's different—diseases and pests which we have to deal with."

How confident are they that they will be able to grow enough? "We're very confident of that," he said. "We've got an expansion program which is going to be hundreds of acres. And we'll be able— ready to meet the demand."

This could be huge, given the obesity epidemic. Phytopharm said it's about to announce marketing plans that will have meal-replacement hoodia products on supermarket shelves by 2008.

MacWilliam said these products are a slightly different species from the hoodia that Stahl tasted in the Kalahari Desert. "It's actually a lot more bitter than the plant that you tasted," said MacWilliam.

The advantage is this species of hoodia will grow a lot faster. But more bitter? How bad could it be? CBS' Leslie Stahl decided to find out. "Not good," she said.

Phytopharm said that when its product gets to market, it will be certified safe and effective. They also promise that it'll taste good.

Buyer Beware

Already, some unscrupulous companies are manufacturing a blend of cheaper ingredients with hoodia claiming that this is better than just hoodia alone. This means that you might find a product containing 1,000 mg of total ingredients, but it may contain as little as 50 mg of hoodia. As a general rule, the other ingredients are only there to make the product cheaper.

All *Hoodia gordonii* supplies worldwide are the same strength. The stems of the plant are picked, dried, and milled. The powder left is about 5 percent of its original weight, which is why some quote a 20:1 extract. But don't be misled. Despite what the label may lead you to believe, you're only getting 50 mg of hoodia.

The minimum dosage to have a usable effect is around 800 to 1,200 mg (that's 800 to 1,200 mg of actual hoodia, whether you call it dried or 20:1 extract). This will help to reduce your appetite (rather than suppress it completely) so you can eat smaller meals and thus lose weight.

If you're interested in trying hoodia, look for a product that has been naturally extracted and grown or ethically wild crafted without the use of chemical fertilizers, pesticides, or preservatives, preferably in a vegetarian capsule. Be sure it is a true standardized full-spectrum herbal supplement without fillers, binders, or common allergens.

Keep in mind that while safety reports to date are encouraging, no large long-term safety studies have been performed. Also, there is no data on possible drug interactions.

Hoodia is a non-stimulating herb, making it more suitable for a broader range of people, since herbal stimulants—caffeine-containing herbs such as guarana or kola nut—can cause side effects such as elevated heart rate and blood pressure, nervousness, and sleeplessness. P57 has no sedative effects.

Waist Management

Losing weight and maintaining an ideal weight requires changing both attitudes and lifestyle. A television advertisement for another weight-loss product depicts people who have used the product successfully bragging about how they lost weight without changing anything about their eating habits and shunning exercising. Let's be real. If your main goal is to quickly lose weight so you can fit into your bathing suit, I have bad news—you may be lighter in weight, but without exercise you're still going to look flabby.

Even though the subjects in the hoodia clinical study did not exercise, you should. Exercise plays an important role in losing and managing weight and in overall health.

Plus, weight loss should be about your overall health. Without proper eating habits, especially nutrition and exercise, you're not accomplishing much. While it's true that less weight puts less stress on your cardiovascular system, you need exercise to strengthen your heart muscles. Proper nutrition and exercise also help prevent many other health problems, including warding off many digestive ailments. (For further information, see Woodland Publishing's *The Good Digestion Guide: A Complete Handbook to Gastrointestinal Health and Happiness.*)

If you want to try hoodia for weight loss, experts suggest supplementing with 800 to 1,200 mg of hoodia a day, divided into two doses and taken with water. Your best bet is to follow the manufacturer's dosage instructions since products may vary. For best results, you should follow a reduced-calorie diet of natural, unprocessed foods. Although you would probably lose weight on a diet like this without supplementing with hoodia, the addition of hoodia may help you stick to your diet better.

The Truth about Low-Carb Diets

A new study shows that almost half of low-carbohydrate dieters believe cutting carbohydrates from their meals is such a magic bullet for weight loss that there is no reason to count calories too. The study, conducted by RoperASW for Slim-Fast Foods Co., included a survey of one thousand adults and two hundred primary-care physicians.

According to the researchers, many people who follow the low-carb craze—which is dying by the way—are in "calorie denial." And doctors say that attitude doesn't bode well for long-term weight loss success. They stress that calories are what count.

"Americans are under tremendous pressure to lose weight," Dr. John Foreyt, a clinical psychologist and director of the Behavioral Medicine Research Center at Baylor College of Medicine, said in a news release announcing the survey results. "As a result, people are willing to believe what defies science—the notion that cutting carbs without cutting calories will generate lasting weight loss. The reality is, it is still important to control calories when following a low-carb diet or any other type of diet."

The survey asked some interesting questions and got some interesting answers:

Q. Do calories matter when you're going low-carb?
A. Forty-six percent of low-carb dieters say they can lose weight by just cutting out the carbs without cutting calories. Fully 86 percent of doctors disagree.

Q. Can you lose weight and keep it off without cutting calories?
A. Fifty-two percent say they can lose weight without cutting calories as long as they restrict carbohydrates. The vast majority of doctors (76 percent) say a diet will only be successful over the long haul if calories are cut, too.

Q. Does portion control matter when you are going low-carb?
A. Thirty-four percent say there is no need to control portion size, while 83 percent of doctors say it is extremely or very important to

do so. Sixty-one percent of doctors are concerned that their patients following a low-carb diet are not controlling their portion sizes as well.

Q. Should people following a low-carb diet worry about getting all the essential nutrients their body needs?
A. Fifty-five percent say there is no worry about getting all the essential nutrients just because carbohydrates are reduced, compared with 95 percent of doctors who note how important it is to get essential nutrients when following this kind of restricted diet.

The researchers say the best advice, no matter what type of diet you're on, is to eat smart. Eat only when you're hungry and don't overeat.

Ways to Spot a Dangerous Diet Plan

This section is specifically addressed to women, since studies show that about half the women in the United States are dieting on any given day. And while they may be successfully losing weight, they could also be on the path to osteoporosis by losing bone density and increasing their risk of fractures and other problems.

Researchers at Rutgers University in New Jersey say that of the eleven most popular weight-loss programs, about half do not contain enough calcium and other critical nutrients, reports FitCommerce.com.

"Women who follow calcium-poor diet plans for extensive periods of time could be causing irreversible damage to their bones and putting themselves at greater risk for osteoporosis," said study coauthor Audrey Cross, Ph.D., faculty member at Rutgers University and author of *Nutrition for the Working Woman*. "Some of the popular diet regimens reinforce the myth that dairy foods are fattening, but any plan that restricts milk and does not provide adequate amounts of calcium may be causing more harm than good."

The top five diets with the least amount of calcium are:

- Dr. Atkins' Diet Revolution
- Sugar Busters
- Suzanne Somers' Fast & Easy
- The Perricone Prescription
- Body for Life

If you follow any of these diets, you'll get less than 60 percent of the daily recommendation for calcium. While women who are nineteen to fifty years old need 1,000 mg of calcium every day, some diets provide as little as 475 mg.

Cross warns women to look for five signs of a dangerous diet:

- It promises a quick fix.
- It lists "good" and "bad" foods.
- It blames specific nutrients or hormones for weight problems.
- It promotes food combining and rigid rules for eating.
- It eliminates one or more food group.

Another recent study showed that people who stop eating dairy products could have a harder time losing weight. A recent study from the Nutrition Institute at the University of Tennessee at Knoxville that was published in the *Journal of Nutrition* concluded that low-fat dairy products may help control body fat. Lead researcher Michael Zemel, Ph.D., professor and head of Tennessee's Department of Nutrition, said that a diet rich in low-fat dairy foods will change the way the body's fat cells do their job. "A diet high in low-fat dairy causes fat cells to make less fat and turns on the machinery to break down fat, which translates into a significantly lower risk of obesity," he explained in a news release announcing the study results. In other words, dairy foods burn fat.

Women seem to benefit the most. "What we found is that women who consumed at least three servings of low-fat dairy foods per day were at the lowest risk of becoming obese," said Zemel. "In fact, there was an 80 percent reduction in risk for any given level of calorie intake."

It's tempting to cut out the dairy foods when we want to lose weight, but when you do this, Zemel says it sends a signal to your body to conserve calcium, which in turn creates higher levels of the hormone calcitriol. It's calcitriol that triggers the production of fat cells. When calcitriol levels are boosted, fat cells expand and store themselves in the body. Translation: You get fat. But when you eat dairy foods, you get more calcium. And calcium suppresses the calcitriol. That in turn breaks down more fat.

All you really need to do is drink two glasses of fat-free milk daily. That will keep your calorie count in check and boost your metabolism.

Fear of the Yo-Yo Effect

Experts agree that the fear of regaining lost pounds is no reason not to lose them in the first place. However, while losing weight is a good idea, repeatedly losing and regaining weight places significant strains on the body—including a woman's immune system, as a recent study at the Fred Hutchinson Cancer Research Center in Seattle, Washington, demonstrates.

According to Cornelia M. Ulrich, Ph.D., senior author and assistant member of the Hutchinson Center's Public Health Sciences Division, weight cycling (the medical term for yo-yo dieting) leads to reduced activity of natural killer cells, which normally destroy viruses and may also have a role in fighting cancer. The more often a woman loses and regains weight, the lower her natural killer cell function becomes and the higher the risk of disease.

In the study, researchers interviewed 114 overweight but otherwise healthy women over age fifty and recorded their weight histories for the past twenty years. Nearly three-quarters of the women had lost more than 10 pounds at least once during that period through dieting. Next, Dr. Ulrich and her colleagues measured the number of the women's natural killer cells via blood tests.

They found that women who lost and regained weight most often—five-plus times over the twenty year period—had the fewest natural killer cells. Also, women who maintained the same weight for five or more years had 40 percent greater natural killer cell activity than those whose weight remained stable for less than two years.

Although the study included only women and further research is needed, Dr. Ulrich believes that the immune systems of men would most likely respond to weight cycling in the same way.

Does this mean it's better to stay overweight? No, says Dr. Ulrich. She says that among those who are obese or overweight, reduced weight has indisputable health benefits. Dr. Ulrich recommends a balanced approach to losing weight. Don't try fad diet after fad diet—that behavior is doomed to failure. Instead, lifestyle change is the cornerstone of weight control. The secret to taking pounds off and keeping them off is to make gradual changes in diet and exercise that you can live with for the rest of your life.

References

"African Plant May Help Fight Fat," CBS News *60 Minutes*, November 23, 2004.

Ahima, R. S. and Osei, S. Y., "Molecular regulation of eating behavior: new insights and prospects for therapeutic strategies," *Trends in Molecular Medicine*, 7, 205–213 (2001).

Bouchard C., Perusse L., "Genetic aspects of obesity," *Annals of the New York Academy of Sciences*, 1993; 699: 26–35.

"The Anti-Fat Pill and the Bushmen," ABC TV, August 25, 2003.

Habeck, Martina, "A succulent cure to end obesity," *Drug Discovery Today*, March 1, 2002; 7(5): 280–281.

MacLean D. B., Luo L-G. "Increased ATP content/production in the hypothalamus may be a signal for energy sensing of satiety: studies of the anorectic mechanism of a plant steroidal glycoside." *Brain Research* 2004; 1020: 1–11.

Mangold, Tom, "Sampling the Kalahari cactus diet," BBC2 News, May 30, 2003.

National Center for Health Statistics, Centers for Disease Control. Prevalence of Overweight among Children and Adolescents: United States, 1999.

Serdula, M. K., Ivery, D., Coates, R. J., et al., "Do obese children become obese adults? A review of the literature," *Preventive Medicine*, 1993; 22: 167–177.

Thompson G., "Bushmen squeeze money from a humble cactus," *The New York Times*, April 1, 2003.

Tulp O. L., Harbi N. A., Mihalov J., DerMarderosian A., "Effect of Hoodia plant on food intake and body weight in lean and obese LA/Ntul//-cp rats," *FASEB* Journal, March 7, 2001, Vol. 15, No. 4, A404.

Tulp, Orien Lee; Harbi, Nevin A. 2002. "Hoodia species as a source of essential micronutrients." *FASEB* Journal, Vol. 16, No. 4, March 20, 2002, A654.

Tulp, Orien Lee; Harbi, Nevin A.; DerMarderosian, Ara, "Effect of Hoodia plant on weight loss in congenic obese LA/Ntul//-cp rats." FASEB Journal, March 20, 2002, Vol. 16, No. 4, A648.

Van Heerden F. R., Vleggaar R., Horak R. M., Learmonth R. A., Maharaj V., Whittal R. D., "Pharmaceutical compositions having appetite suppression activity," United States Patent 6,376,657, issued April 23, 2002.

Whitaker, R. C., Wright, J. A., Pepe, M. S., Seidel, K. D., Dietz, W. H., "Predicting obesity in young adulthood from childhood and parental obesity," *New England Journal of Medicine*, 1997; 337: 869–873.